The Holy Movement: Matters Of The Colon

© 2000 by Debora Lee Meehan

Published by:
New Century Press
1055 Bay Boulevard, Suite C
Chula Vista, CA 91911
(800) 519-2465
(619) 476-7400
www.newcenturypress.com
E-mail: sales@newcenturypress.com

Library of Congress Card Number: 00-108752
ISBN 1-890035-19-X

COVER DESIGN BY NEW CENTURY PRESS

10 9 8 7 6 5 4 3 2 1

Mission Statement

My mission is to teach others that it's our God-given right, privilege and responsibility to exercise the principle of stewardship of the temple, which is your mind, body, and soul life. God has devised at conception by innate ability for you to understand how to appropriately use the resources in nature to restore health to your mind, body, and soul. Whenever trauma has befallen mind, body or soul, you have been given access to total restoration, in order that you may enjoy a full, rich, and abundant life.

Benediction

As 1999 was coming to an end, I realized that I couldn't continue into the next century without committing the last 14 years of my life and studies to paper. I was having difficulty sleeping at night with an endless dialogue of healing stories. Of course, after checking out all the physical possibilities of insomnia, I realized that sleep wouldn't come easily until I birthed this verbal baby. Besides, my neck will finally get thinner as soon as I do this.

To my fellow human beings please accept my gift and contribution to you for the new century.

May these words of truth penetrate and permeate every level of cell and tissue of your mind, body and soul.

Dedication

This book is written with dedication and honor to my Aunt Beryl in appreciation of her love, guidance and inspiration, with passion, to achieve success in our life times.

It's with great pleasure I also dedicate this book to my daughter, Lauren, my son, Jamie, and my husband, Kevin.

To my children, I'm eternally thankful for having the awesome privilege of raising them. For it was in their childrearing that I became truly whole. It's hard to believe those days are over, leaving precious memories that I'll always cherish. My children are my greatest assets, and it's through them I've greatly manifested success. Their wonderfully generous, loving lives are a great contribution to this world now and will be in the future. They both will be instrumental in the healing arts, as they continue to walk circumspectly through life.

To my husband, Kevin, I dedicate this book for his great example of what unconditional love is and how energizing it can be when given freely. He's the greatest example of this love that I've ever known in my lifetime. For his love I'm eternally thankful. I know that I've been loved and that the curses of the fathers have been broken by deliberate decision of my children and my husband and myself. Our family and generations to come will live in truth and love.

Gratitude to Others

I owe many thanks to the following people who with their contributions have led me to the truth and the abundant life. May God bless your hearts and souls for your gift ministries that have proven helpful for the perfecting of the Saints! And to all the people with whom I came in contact who may not have realized they were being inspired to give me the specific information that I happened to be seeking at that moment.

Dr. Hulda Clark, Ph.D., N.D., *"The Cure for All Diseases"*

Dr. Larry Crab, *"Inside Out"*

John Bradshaw, *"The Family" and "Healing the Shame That Binds You"*

Mechtchild Scheffer, *"Bach Flower Therapy"*

Dr. Peter J. D'Adamo with Catherine Whitney, *"Eat Right for Your Type"*

Ann Wigmore, *"The Wheat Grass Book"*

Suzanne White, *"The New Astrology"*

University Medical Research Publishers, *"Amazing Medicines the Drug Companies Don't Want You to Discover"*

Caroline Myss, Ph.D., *"Anatomy of the Spirit"*

John Robbins, *"Diet for A New America"*

Dr. Bernard Jensen, *"Tissue Cleansing Through Bowel Management"*

The Diamonds, *"Fit for Life"*

Rick Pitino, *"Success Is A Choice"*

Ted J. Kaptchuk, O.M.D., *"The Web That Has No Weaver"*

George Anderson, *"We Do Not Die"* and *"We Are Not Forgotten"*
Rev. George Malkmus, *"Why Christians Get Sick"*
Joseph and Helen Wood, *Wood Hygienic Institute*
Dr. Kristen Nicol, NET, *Biochemical and Bach Flower Therapies*
Cindy Moonrose, *Energy Work, Intuitive Counseling*
Dr. John Upledger, *Cranial Sacral Therapy*
Marc Anthony, *When I Dream at Night Album, Heart Chakra Therapy*
Angie Dee, *Neuromuscular Therapy*

Contents

CHAPTER 1

The Stewardship Principle

The simple reality is sometimes difficult for us to see and often seems to be quite a challenge for us. But the ultimate responsibility lies within us individually; it'll always be that way in truth. Basically history always states it to be that way. I Corinthians 3:16-18 states:

> *Know Ye Not That Ye Are The Temple Of God And That The Spirit Of God Dwelleth In You? If Any Man Defile The Temple Of God, Him Shall God Destroy; For The Temple Of God Is Holy, Which Temple Ye Are.*

So maybe you can't pray to God for certain aspects of our health, because he designed that we solely have that responsibility. In the physical plane it is spiritual to keep your body clean internally and externally. Maybe as a culture, we've forgotten those simple aspects of health, life, and spirituality. There appears to be a sowing and reaping slant to this when God says, *"If any man defile the temple of God, him shall God destroy..."* So I guess asking God to heal you because you ate two pies in two days and now you're sick would be out of the question. So at what point does ignorant bliss suffice for innocence? Of course, we can stay ignorant or choose to become enlightened.

1

I do believe Reverend George Malkmus has done a commendable job of informing the public of the Biblical and historical information involving diets and their connection with life spans throughout history. His book is titled, *Why Christians Get Sick.*

CHAPTER 2

Receive, Retain, Release Principle

I first learned this principle from the Bible, James 1:21. God tells us to receive the Word with meekness and that it's able to save our souls. We must retain it with conviction, by being doers of that work, not just hearers only, or we're deceiving ourselves. Release the word with boldness, so the spoken truth will set others free. As others in turn practice this principle, they become doers of the word. The reward is stated in verse 25 "… this man shall be blessed in his deed."

I deliberately set out to change my life. In 1976, I started applying spiritual laws or principles to accomplish this change. In 1987, it became obvious that I'd not be able to complete my physical life here on earth unless I started to obey these principles many have before: Dr. Bernard Jensen, Dr. Norman Walker, Jason Winters, and many more. In fact, if you research historically, you'll practice the receive, retain, release principle in the daily stewardship of your digestive tract. First I realized that I'd have to take the accumulative garbage of 30 years out of my large intestine. The process was simple: I just thought of how I'd clean my house and followed those innate impulses. I did 7-day colon cleansing programs that I researched from many sources. Then I implemented these programs and delivered the dead old feces that were stealing my energy. Immediately my energy levels increased and my body began to heal. I continued this program for six years.

Wisdom is knowledge applied! Remember knowledge isn't effective unless it's applied. It's uncanny how much research people will do without application of this research, and somehow think they've become experts. As James says in I: 22, "deceiving your own selves." When bowel cleansing is done properly, you'll always gain positive results. The quality of my life is evidence, just as there've been many before: Dr. Bernard Jensen, Dr. Norman Walker, Jason Winters, and many more. If you research historically you'll find almost every culture back to 4000 B.C. did practice colon hygiene as a regular modality for maintaining good health. This is simply natural internal hygiene.

CHAPTER 3

The Gall of the Matter

A consistent student of bowel management was beginning to have some severe gallbladder problems. This man had been in the electronic end of the music business during the 1980's in the Los Angeles area. During this period he was under much stress, spent long laborious hours of intense physical labor and serious partying!

Now in the mid-nineties he needed to pay his physical debt back to his body. He aggressively worked on his bowel management but was becoming burdened with sleepless nights because of gallbladder spasms. Without rest he'd soon hit bottom. We discussed his situation, and I suggested the idea of cleansing his liver and gallbladder with a simple little flush. I shared with him my success from flushing my liver and gallbladder and suggested that it might help his situation. Up until this point I was the only person I knew that had experimented with this flush. But he realized he had nothing to lose.

The only other option was to have his gallbladder surgically removed. Living without an organ, in my opinion, isn't an easy alternative. God designed the body wonderfully and perfectly, with every organ uniquely designed for its specific contribution to the whole body's wellness. It was time for him to make a decision. So for a small amount of time and money he chose to do the flush. Though you initially feel a little nauseated, it's a small price to pay for wellness. He released many gallstones into his toilet at home and followed up with a colonic at mid-day. His body released hundreds of small green or cholesterol stones and hundreds of calcified stones through the colonic tube. Really surprising to me, but since then I've seen this many times over, was the size of the calcified stones. They were consistently the size of a quarter! Hundreds of them! HOLY CRAP! Of course he admitted to having taken, over the last ten years, pack after pack of Rolaids and Tums, which are consistent with the content of these stones. Needless to say, this man was feeling good. Sleepless nights turned into sleep-full nights.

I'd like to mention at this time some interesting observations having to do with this subject. First, everyone who has done a flush has passed at least hundreds of stones. Even people who have had their gallbladders removed have passed stones. Hulda Clark's book, *"Cure for All Diseases,"* discusses in detail this flushing process. I've seen some stones as large as a golf ball. The first flush usually will contain a lot of small stones with a lot of chaff. The second flush will usually contain larger stones. It appears that the gallbladder and liver will innately open up easier after the first flush, almost like priming. Also, I've known people to do these flushes and not release any stones, but with a colonic, will pass them. Obviously, their bowel must be too full for the stones to move out easily. Flushing our organs may prove to be an easy and powerful tool for gaining our health and continuing to keep us on the path to wellness.

CHAPTER 4

The Tapeworm Story-Tenant Eviction

It was June 1997 when I received a phone call from a woman in Murfreesboro. She'd been ill for 11 years and told me she'd come to the end of her rope, so to speak. She said that she'd prayed and told God that she'd do whatever it took to get well. It's always a little scary for me when people say these kinds of things to me, because when someone has asked God for guidance and wisdom, they are going to get just that. How I fit into this equation is a mystery unfolding. When she came into my office she told me that she'd never driven outside of Murfreesboro, and that it was a miracle she found my office.

By this time her family and close friends were tired and frustrated with her health dilemma. She felt alone and afraid. Many years ago she was diagnosed with abnormal stomach bacteria and for some reason, allowed her surgeon to remove her uterus and ovaries, having two partial hysterectomies throughout an 11-year period. With absolutely no change in her condition, she obviously continued her search for wellness. She stated her symptoms as follows: An enormous appetite; never getting complete satisfaction with the amount or choice of food; feeling tired always, not even wanting to get out of bed; experiencing low energy levels; and feeling ready to give up. As far as her appearance went, she looked healthy, bio-chemically speaking; her face displayed no obvious deficiencies or clues to her illness. She was in my opinion a little on the thin side. She also mentioned at this time that she'd started taking barley green several months ago: 1 tablespoon 4 times per day. And for some reason, a foul odor was coming from her body cavity, and her family was complaining about it.

So she decided to do a 15 colonic series, doing consecutive colonics, 5 days on, 2 off, until the 15 were completed. Her body released a lot of florescent drugs, probably from the surgeries, and small worms. We also saw flat square sections of a tapeworm passing through the acrylic tube. I asked her in the middle of the series if she'd be willing to try something that I learned from Dr. Bernard Jensen's book. If you starve a tapeworm for a couple days by not eating, it'll become so hungry that if you sit over a pan of warm milk and honey, it'll travel through the colon and out the anus in pursuit of the milk. She agreed, bless her heart! When we did the process, there was no response. We even held the honey jar up at her mouth, as tapeworms are also known to chase food that way, but still nothing happened. In reviewing some information concerning the odor present along with the fact that she'd taken barley green for several months consistently, we concluded that it was dead already and decaying. From previous research, I learned that the only way to kill a tapeworm is by ingesting large amount of digestive enzymes for long periods of time, which allows the enzymes to digest the head of the tapeworm so it cannot grow its body again. Barley green is a fabulous source of enzymes.

As her series came to an end, I felt we'd paved a passageway for the tapeworm to journey from her stomach to her colon, and then to exit her anus, knowing her body would perform the release process beautifully. To help this process, I asked her to consistently take her cleansing herbs and to do at least 3 enemas per week.

If there was ever a faithful person, she was it. I heard from this wonderful woman in mid-September. She was somewhat distraught because she hadn't passed any fecal matter even with an enema for 9 days. Now, she felt a large ball passing across her transverse colon and it was quite painful. I simply reminded her of her prayer to God stating that she'd do anything to get well, and that He'd not bring her to this place and time to abandon her. I told her that her body was doing a great job transporting this unwanted tenant out the door. Her body just needed some help. I exhorted her to take a coffee enema, as it would provide her parasalstis with the stimulation necessary to kick the worm completely out. And that's exactly what happened. She called me in the morning and said it was like delivering a small baby. Four thirty-inch pieces exited her body. The water was dark from the coffee, and she almost flushed the toilet without taking a sample. Thank God she took a utensil and pulled the proof out of the toilet! Her husband who happened to be a farmer, when seeing it said, "It looks like a tapeworm"! So I traveled down to Murfreesboro to witness this parasite and brought it back to my office to show my clients what a tapeworm looked like.

One thing I forgot to mention: When this woman started out, she had a look in her eyes that I'd never seen before, an expression of total fear as if she'd seen a ghost. I thought that look was strange, but did not understand until the tapeworm was gone. Now the expression in her eyes was one of peace and tranquility.

One year later I received another phone call from her. She was passing the same size pieces of the tapeworm again. I told her that there is always a family. Research says that tapeworms are asymptomatic*, which means in most cases they live harmoniously with their carrier and that every other person has a tapeworm! I suppose this woman was claiming her territory and her health back by cleaning her temple with simple natural internal hygiene. And we all said, "HOLY CRAP!"

*asymptomatic – Some species of tapeworms have become so well adapted to life in the human body, that the host (man) may be entirely asymptomatic.

This means you may have a tapeworm and <u>not</u> appear to have any symptoms. You wouldn't even know it was there."The Essentials of Medical Parasitology" by Thomas J. Brooks Jr., M. D.

CHAPTER 5

Psychic Healing

One extraordinary story I'll always remember is this one. It was August 1998. A woman called me who had had a colonic two years previously and I remembered her clearly. She was a psychic in the Nashville area. She told me that as she was reading her Tarot cards concerning an engagement in the month of November, still two months away, the cards read that she was deceased. After digesting this horrible news, she sought out her health care practitioner of choice to check her health status. The prognosis was grim, as her liver was barely functioning. She decided to do consecutive colonics. After one month of colonics she asked me what my opinion was on her having 2 colonics per day. I told her the story of the girl who needed a liver transplant, and that certainly several colonics per day served to be useful in her recovery. She decided to do 2 per day. Through the months of September and October she did 2 colonics per day.

At this time she also researched information concerning the cleansing of certain organs. Having already successfully cleansed my own liver, gallbladder, and pancreas, I helped her execute these valuable procedures. She flushed out many gallstones, which Hulda Clark states in her book,

15

"Cure for All Diseases," the stones come basically from the liver. So doing these flushes certainly helps detox the bacteria and viruses as well as the stones through the duodenum into the intestines and then exit the body through the anus. It's important at this point to discuss the rebuilding of the systems and organs. When you do intense cleansing, it's important to do intense rebuilding, in order to supply the body with the proper fuel to rebuild and heal. This woman was well educated in the supplemental aspects of health. As well as whole food supplements, she took bovine glandular, which are excellent for energizing the endocrine system. She also felt it necessary to support her thyroid gland.

November came and went, and she saw much improvement in her health. She also researched diet and nutrition, utilizing the book, *"Eat Right for Your Type."* She began a high-protein diet, consisting of fish and eggs, a little fruit, sticking with an enzymatic fruit such as pineapple, lots of green vegetables, and almost no starch. Again she saw more improvement. Another important key to recovery is a lot of rest. As this woman will attest to, if you're not willing to be kind enough to your body and give it proper amounts of rest, the body will simply take the time and you just have to accept that. She's still on her path to wellness as we all are, thankful to have received and applied this wealth of knowledge. And we all said, "HOLY CRAP!"

CHAPTER 6

It Was 1999 and My Daughter…

It was 1999 and my daughter, Lauren, was going into the spring of her senior year of high school. I decided it was time for her to do the most important thing she could do for herself and that was to clean up her environment. Time for her to do her first colonic series. Although she was nervous, but being the Taurus she is, stayed faithful to her schedule of 5 colonics per week until they were completed.

Lauren had no major illness or health problems. The only problem was that she had developed approximately 35 warts of various types. Two of them were planters' warts on the bottom of her feet that were becoming very uncomfortable.

So we completed the series of colonics and within 5 days, all her warts dried up and fell off. HOLY CRAP! So if warts are caused by a virus in the blood, then cleaning up her bowel led to cleaning up her blood.

CHAPTER 7

The Worm Story

It was 1993, and I was about to learn a lot more of what was involved in the exploration of colon hygiene.

A 25-year-old woman from Pennsylvania came to my office. Her doctors had diagnosed her with Epstein-Barr virus (EBV) or the herpes virus that causes mononucleosis (commonly known as the "kissing disease"), advanced hepatitis, and chronic fatigue. She was told her only hope was a liver transplant, but she refused that idea. She was on her deathbed and her family was mourning for her soon-to-be death. She said that Jesus Christ appeared to her along with some angels and they told her she would not die. Somehow she hooked up with my good friend who had become a N.D., or naturopathic doctor, in Philadelphia. So my friend called and asked if they could fly to my office and possibly we could help this woman. Of course, was my answer.

I listed her diagnoses and noticed also that she was quite frail and weak, pretty much confined to bed and a wheelchair. Her health had slowly deteriorated over the last 10 years, at which time she'd done hard drugs and alcohol for 3 or 4 years straight. Now facing an emaciated body and devastating future, she was willing to try anything to get well.

My friend, the N.D., had studied with a group of doctors who were practicing more of an Eastern type of healthcare, along the lines of bringing the body into balance by correcting the three sides within the body of healing: emotional, structural, and bio-chemical. She was using contact reflex analysis to keep her body balanced nutritionally, and at this point, that was a miracle in itself. Remember, this woman's liver wasn't working, she couldn't eat food with the exception of chewing and spitting out the food repeatedly, only to chew and gain some nutrition from the chewing, and swallowing the saliva only, never the food itself.

She only muscle-tested for 3 foods: brown rice, papaya, and pineapple. Also she was taking whole food complexes from the Standard Process line of supplements, which were keeping her body nutritionally supported.

So now it was time for her to have some colonics. She muscle-tested for 4 per day. After each colonic was finished she'd have great amounts of energy and within 3 hours would be almost delirious. The first colonic was quite an eye-opener for me because at this point in my career, I really didn't know that parasites existed at the level they did. Through the acrylic tube I saw worms that looked like large night crawlers. And not just a few but hundreds packed together going through the tube. HOLY CRAP! I COULD NOT BELIEVE MY EYES!

Then Dr. Nicol said, "Look at those suckers, they're worms!" That was only the beginning. For 8 days, 4 times per day we saw nothing but worms, worms, and more worms. Also any fecal matter that passed through the tube was snow-white, indicating that her liver had shut down.

After 8 days of wonderful learning bliss Dr. Nicol and our client flew home to Philadelphia. Now this woman was daily under Dr. Nicol's care. Along with supporting her body bio-chemically she also gave herself 15 enema bags a day. It was almost like bailing out a sinking boat, as the waste was removed from the bowel. The organs and cells would then fill that vacuum back up in the bowel with more waste that had built up over years in her system. This process repeated itself for days and months.

She returned three more times until the end of January 1994. At the time of her second visit she was having 2 colonics per day for 8 days. Still there were many worms and she muscle-tested for over 50 digestive enzymes a day (digestive enzymes eat up bacteria which parasites are.) At the end of this visit she returned home and was much more energetic. In fact she started driving, which she'd not been physically capable of doing for the past three years. She was also able to eat a few foods, only organic and raw. It was apparent that her liver was starting

21

to work again. Her fecal matter was brown at this point.

As her body was cleaning up its environment, she was muscle-testing for even more foods and was gaining back her strength. She was no longer emaciated or in a wheel chair and was becoming quite active. Her skin was beginning to show a real healthy glow.

Her family was singing praises to the Lord and sending us wonderful cards full of gratitude. And Dr. Nicol and I were just as thankful as they were. To have such an opportunity delivered to us was truly the highest honor I could imagine.

CHAPTER 8

Black Worm Day

Over the last 14 years of practicing colon hygiene perhaps the most interesting and provocative events seem to occur when the individual chooses to do a 15 series of colonics, having a colonic once a day for 5 days, 2 days off, then 5 on, until the 15 are completed. It even becomes more interesting when several people are doing a series on the same schedule. What becomes apparent is the same pattern that develops between the outcomes of these individuals doing the colonics.

During the first 5 to 7 colonics, the bowel will begin to eliminate approximately 2 to 5 times per day on the toilet in addition to having a colonic; this occurs with the help of ingesting cleansing herbs such as cascara, sagrada cactus, fennel, sienna, peppermint, cape aloe, etc. So how can the bowel eliminate so much fecal matter in one day? The answer is simple. The bowel must contain plenty of fecal matter. In fact the bowel is quite willing to accommodate the helpful actions of the colonics and herbs in removing this matter.

It is common knowledge that infants will have a bowel movement within 20 minutes of eating. The feces contained in that bowel movement are from 24 hours previous. What's releasing 20 minutes after breakfast is yesterday's breakfast. It's interesting that the infant will release on schedule until the child starts to eat processed food over and over again. Eventually many of us stop having a bowel movement 20 minutes after we eat as we progress in age. Why? Because the bowel is filling up with waste that cannot exit because the bowel was never designed to eat processed food. There is no memory bank present in the body to handle this situation. The body tries to protect itself by walling off the old feces, storing them as they harden and stick along the wall of the colon. This process is confirmed throughout history by many autopsy doctors and by the outcome of colon hygiene. Almost every person within a period of 3 weeks, staying faithful to the formula, will begin to have a bowel movement within 20 minutes of a meal. The body will begin to be restored to its innate ability to release after a meal, just as it always did early in life. Thus, if colon hygiene helps to restore this innate ability to the body it's proven to be truthful and necessary.

There's a reason for the title of this story: During a colonic series, somewhere between the 5th and 10th colonic, the bowel may consistently release small 1-inch black worms. These appear to be like colonies of hundreds of worms. The release proves to be so consistent that one day during 8 hours of colonics, every person (8 people) released black worms during their colonic. Thus, I designated this day "black worm day"… and we all said, "HOLY CRAP!"

CHAPTER 10

Baby Sitting the Environment

The story's unfolding as I'm writing this book in February of 2000. This unique story I thought would make its own special contribution to internal hygiene and our search for all truth.

My colleague and good friend is having her first child at age 27. It's wonderful to watch a couple at this stage of life, and also remindful for me of those years of my life. The couple is living so vitally " in the moment."

This woman is probably one of only a few alternative health care professionals who really have utilized the modality of colon hygiene for the maximum benefit available throughout her young life. So when she became pregnant, she continued to utilize this modality to ensure a safe and clean environment for her and her baby.

Of course, colonic irrigations should be used during pregnancy ONLY if the woman's been doing colonics routinely before the pregnancy, as was this particular case. This woman had had routine colonics for many years and is presently having 2 to 4 colonics per month. Anyone who practices colon hygiene routinely will know at what pace to move during pregnancy. By this point you've learned to trust your body's ability to communicate with the higher self. My friend's thankful that she understands this modality and is elated to receive the rewards and blessings it's provided to her and her baby during pregnancy. If you asked her to describe her experience, knowing her, she'd probably say, "HOLY CRAP!"

CHAPTER 11

"Perfect Timing"

In early summer of 1998, I received a phone call from a man concerning his father. His father, a Nashville resident, had contracted cancer and the children flew in from around the country to discuss their father's health situation and his options. The young man had practiced colon hygiene in a western state and was a big fan of this particular modality. I realized that he was basically interviewing me and I passed. I explained to him in order to see any improvement in overall energy levels, a person needs to do at least 15 colonics in a 20-day period; otherwise, you may be wasting your time. Also it was important to be supporting the body with some basic nutrition. I was surprised and thankful that his children were knowledgeable about disease and already had him taking those necessary nutritional foods.

The father was in his seventies, and was one of the healthiest people I've ever met and had one of the healthiest bowels I've ever seen! He'd contracted cancer recently because of his new career. He learned a lot about his illness from Dr. Hulda Clark's book, *"Cure for All Diseases."* Educating himself about his health, he moved into empowerment and control of his own life. He did a

15 series of colonics with a short break in the middle and was delighted. I'm always amazed to see the various types of people who come into a serious life crisis and how they innately choose the life-giving modalities to bring back the quality of their life and many times will go beyond. For such wise choices we have a lot to be thankful.

This man promised to call me back with the test results concerning his illness; they were negative and the cancer was gone. And, he'd also learned a lot about the prevention of that illness. One thing I want to share about this particular family is that they really worked together as a family in crisis, handling these challenges, checking out their options, making decisions, each person doing what was necessary. It was nice to see such a cooperative and helping family. And once again we all said, "HOLY CRAP!"

CHAPTER 12

My Biography Is My Biology

Many thanks to Caroline Myss for her contribution, *"Anatomy of the Spirit,"* where she used simple truth to describe simple health: "…Your biography becomes biology…" I've chosen to begin the story of my life's biography with this statement.

Although I've decided to begin at the year 1987, I'll have to set the stage first. Basically, I'm the second oldest of four children, the two eldest being female, the two youngest male. My father was diagnosed with various mental health illnesses that involved him spending much time in the Veterans' hospital during the 1960's and 1970's. My mother was aggressive in her career, secured a good position with a bank during these years and was the provider for our household. She ended her career at retirement and moved to sunny Florida with her husband of 20 years.

My father passed away in a Veterans' hospital in 1990. He'd lived there since 1985 and ultimately died from emphysema. He was born to immigrant Italians in the Norristown, Pennsylvania area during the 1940's and 1950's, one of thirteen children. My mother was the second daughter of four children, born and raised in the countryside of beautiful Chester County just outside of Philadelphia.

At this point, I'd like to acknowledge John Bradshaw's contribution to America. His two books, *"The Family"* and *"Healing the Shame That Binds You"* have exposed the generational emotional disorders that have held human beings in bondage for generations. This information has brought light and understanding to us, enabling us to be set free to experience the more-than-abundant life. Many thanks to this man for his perseverance and integrity in searching for the truth.

CHAPTER 13

The First Lesson in Truth!

This family situation was the first time in my life that I came to the realization that our actions hold the key to the power. It's in the doing of the truth that the positive and permanent changes will come and ultimately change our future. Curses from the fathers are passed down from generation to generation. It's these curses that bring the emotional traumas that trigger the negative neurotransmitters to be transmitted into the organs and tissues of the body that bring about premature degeneration and disease. Working backward would be the way to go. You must search out therapists who know how to do this work. Don't be distracted by thinking these therapists are mainstream. God has set these gift ministries where it pleased Him, not according to the great American culture.

In the late 1970's and early 1980's we were exclusively involved with a Bible organization. We studied the Bible along with the Greek, the Aramaic, the understanding of Eastern customs, and oriental cultures. But most importantly we put much emphasis on the practical application of this information to our daily routines. People considered our lifestyles to be somewhat cultic. But I was open to learning as much as I could about life and truth.

Thank God I had a sponge mentality! At this time I specifically became interested in learning about the family and how to raise my children. I was a young mother and realized that I'd basically raised myself, based on some instinctive survival skills. But those protective skills weren't sound principles for raising children that I was sure of.

My son's early life wasn't an easy one; he experienced his parents' nasty divorce at the age of three, which left him full of fear, hate and anger. He literally became so outraged that he attacked and hit and bit me as much as he could. Many people witnessed this behavior with disbelief that a youngster could have such hostility. Of course, I realized, as I studied the Scriptures, that as the parent, I held the key and the power to the quality of this child's life and that I was willing to accept that full responsibility. The other wonderful thing I learned during these years was that as I taught my children these wonderful truths, I was also learning them myself, so we'd all benefit!

I began to study the Book of Timothy and discovered that the Scriptures were profitable for doctrine, reproof, and correction, which is instruction in righteousness. So that format is what I used to instruct my children in obedience Ephesians 6:1-2 states:

> *Children, obey your parents in the Lord; for this is right. Honor thy father and*

THE FIRST LESSON IN TRUTH!

mother; which is the first commandment with promise;

But let me go back to the fact that the parents need to be in the lord! That doesn't mean that you do everything perfectly or even religiously, but only that you carry out your responsibility of teaching your own children the truths of the Word of God. It's not your church's responsibility, or you're pastor's, or that of the United States of America or the Pope… simply yours. The accountability in our lives always falls on the owner of that particular temple or body.

The blessing PROMISED is in verse 3, *"That it may be well with thee, and thou mayest live long on the earth"*; this is the inspirational part of the message. Such was my wish for my son's life that motivated me to act in accordance with Ephesians 6. My son was heading for a disastrous life. Thank God, being the Virgo I am, that my philosophy's always been if you're going to do anything, do it right, especially when the right tools and instruction are provided by God Almighty. What do you have to lose? The only time we lose is when we make the wrong choices that violate truth. And I'm sure the divine design is so that we're all on a level playing field. No matter what your name is or how much so-called worldly success you've had or how great your possessions are, the more than abundant life is obtainable by human beings who may live anywhere, in any culture, who seek the truth for their lives.

During the early 1980's people who'd witnessed my son's behavior were making quite positive comments about the obvious and wonderful changes in his deep-seated personality. And new acquaintances were telling me that my son was always welcome in their homes because he was a blessing and a wonderful influence on their children. The ultimate promise from Ephesians 6:3, *"That it will be well with thee,"* was literally ringing true.

As my children grew (my son just as I am writing this story made me a grandmother in February 2000, he being 26 years old), many people told me that I was lucky to have two wonderful children. Even though I'd never take their precious lives for granted, I know in my heart of hearts that their lives were ultimately shaped by the truths that we took the time together as a family to learn and apply each and every day. We did as any successful athlete or anybody does to obtain real success in any avenue in life. I do understand there are things in life that are out of our control such as accidental sufferings and Karmic situations, and during those times we can only make the best of such situations.

God does give us specific instruction about many things in our lives over which we have direct and ultimate control and influence and that's where we need to direct our energies and attention. And we must take time to research specifically what those things are. And that research will require work. On the physical plane work will always be required. And we are body, soul, and spirit beings. Physical plane work is a spiritual work. Just praying for your life to change in any category requires work of some sort. Why would we think that we should just be able to pray for good health, as we sit on our butts popping all kinds of polluted foods and sugary-sweet drinks into our bodies? Not to mention all the legal drugs people are pouring into their bodies because a so-called expert, who happens to be another ignorant human being, tells you it's O.K. to do. It's your challenge and responsibility for your own benefit to take the time to love yourself enough to pursue and study ALL the information out there, which will enable you to make better decisions.

Remember it's your God-given right to make your own choices, nobody else's, good or bad. Your actions will ultimately dictate the outcome. God shouldn't be blamed for our self-inflicted ignorance and poor choices. We're only kidding ourselves with our intellectual egos, lives filled with less quality and spinning out of control into early graves. Call it old-fashioned but if simplicity's old-fashioned, then I'm there. No matter how much technology we obtain, we're still organic and will always fare better with organic substances, you can never top that. People thousands of years ago were far healthier and superior, and their technology wasn't shabby, either. Check out those pyramids! If you check out ancient civilizations, you'll find consistent practicing of herbs and colon hygiene. Colon hygiene's not a fad or a new idea; it's as old as the earth, which makes it prophetic by nature. It's simply old information coming to a new generation.

CHAPTER 14

1987

In March 1987 my daughter, Lauren, my husband of seven years, and myself, moved to Nashville. My son, Jamie, was fourteen years old and was living with his father in Pennsylvania. Leaving the Bible College and relocating here, we found ourselves in a good position financially; we'd been out of debt for five years. Lucky for me, because it was quite obvious that I was very ill. I slept nearly sixteen hours a day, barely had the energy to go to the grocery store. When I did go out, I was exhausted. I had neck and back problems. My neck was out of alignment as a -11, a healthy neck would be a +17. I had pain in all my tissue and joints and felt very old. I was displaying symptoms of Lupus and fibromyalgia.*

Although back in 1987 little was known or addressed concerning both of these health situations.

I was doing bowel management, learned and started while at the Bible College. Some people in the program were vegetarians and gave me information on various methods to accomplish this task. Twice a year I did do a colon cleanse that consisted of this: for 7 days; psyllium seed 4x per day; bennonite 4x per day; mix both together with distilled water, drink 4x per day; no food for 7 days.

Lupus is severe inflammation throughout many areas of the body; fibromyalagia is aching and stiffness in muscles.

My nutritional source was green magma, 24 tablets per day, ending each day with a coffee enema for those 7 days.

I carried out this procedure every 6 months from 1987 to 1992, and was quite happy with the results. About 3 days into the cleanse, I began to feel better than ever, my energy levels would soar, my eyes would get clear, and the serious spinal problems in my neck and back almost disappeared. Understanding that the toxins were literally detoxing out of my spinal column within days of the start of a cleanse truly exhilarated me. I was on to an important piece of the puzzle of healthcare.

During these times I recollected memories that as a child I never had energy. My endurance levels were not what they should've been for a child, because of being athletic and outgoing, when I complained of not feeling well, nobody believed me. I was both mentally and physically fatigued. My attention span was short. From the waist down I was immaturely developing, my upper body did not match my lower body visually or strength wise. As I reached puberty, twice a month for a day period I would get a migraine headache and go blind in one eye; this happened until I started to menstruate. Of course, the doctor said this was normal, although I knew of no one else who had these troubles during puberty.

In 1987 bowel management gave me some hope of feeling well. With my research, I realized there were many other health issues that needed to be addressed in order to gain my full health. I won't say, "gain back," because I'd never had good health to begin with. This realization motivated me to search for the whole truth concerning the bio-chemical, structural, and emotional sides of healing. I wanted it all. I was determined to secure the abundant life by my own actions, taking time to love myself enough to clean and nurture the internal parts of my body.

CHAPTER 15

1992

It is 1992. Did you ever wonder when things would slow down some? There are periods of time when you go rapidly through many changes that bring you to a whole new place in life. This was one of those times, in the middle of an eleven-year marriage that was ending in divorce. I needed to make some career decisions. I left the hair industry and flew to the Helen Wood Institute in Florida to study with her.

This was my fifth year of practicing bowel management on myself, and simultaneously many doors opened in this direction. I realized that this modality was a beneficial tool for my own recovery. It was during these years my household practiced routine bowel management. My dear friend, Dr. Nicol, visited every 6 to 8 weeks, both of us starting out in our fields, she in naturopathy and of course I was the expert in environmental clean-up.

I remarried in 1993 and fortunately for my husband and myself, health was an important issue to both of us. Kevin was thrilled to be practicing bowel management. My son, Jamie, who was 19 at that time, also was in pursuit of environmental cleanup and we did clean his total bowel in less than three years. During these three years, Dr. Nicol,

Kevin, Jamie, myself and anybody who had the good fortune to visit and participate had changed the course of their lives. I consider those years a vital part of my education. We all were live laboratory rats, in a perfect position for learning and documenting research in this field of colon hygiene. We explored our bodies and our boundaries with this modality, only to find abundant benefits.

At this time Dr. Nicol was also taking care of us with bio-chemical and neurological emotional analysis. At this point, we were all groovin' and movin' diligently in full triangular motion, gaining much healing structurally, bio-chemically and emotionally.

I've included documentation of my bowel management (see Chapter 19) starting in 1987. By 1992, I replaced the 7-day colon cleansing and fasting program with colonics. I entered my 6th and 7th years of bowel management, moving aggressively. Considering how dynamic I was feeling, I was willing to see and learn all that truth would teach me. I allowed my body to teach me and subjected my bowel management regimen according to how my body felt, instead of according to the comments and opinions of people who'd never attempted any bowel management.

It finally occurred to me that I was traveling into unexplored territory with the exception of Dr. Bernard Jensen, Dr. Norman Walker and a few others. All the healing and beneficial changes were occurring in my body and health, just as I was witnessing all the types of old hardened feces and parasites leaving my body cavity, as all these doctors explained in their books. I used the correct tool, in the correct manner, for the correct amount of time, and therefore the outcome was the same for all of us. If someone doesn't use this modality correctly they'll not get the same results. It would be like trying to saw a large tree down with a small hacksaw. This is where common sense comes in.

I want to convey to you at this time the importance of taking the proper supplements. When doing bowel management, it's important to understand that you'll deplete some valuable minerals in your body. The body will begin to heal from the poison exiting from the body. You want to rebuild with some good flora support and other whole food complexes. I utilized contact reflex analysis as my diagnostic tool to ensure proper supplementation, and thus learned what my bio-chemical health challenges were for my unique makeup. Having learned these changes, I didn't need to continue my search for that particular bit of information. It was time to be faithful to carrying out this procedure by taking what I needed as I continued to clean the poison out of my body. It was amazing how well the organic supplements worked on my clean body.

As my body reaped the benefits of cleansing and fueling with organic food, it was prime time to continue my emotional work. When the mind, body, and soul are in rhythm with the innate understanding of the process to receive, retain, release, and then you create fertile ground to let the emotions release easily. The muscle memory to release is getting exercised over and over and over again, and the body will begin to do this at the drop of a hat.

You've retrained your body to recognize when you want to let go.

It was at this time that I released the issue of abandonment from my 2nd and 3rd charkas, located in the abdominal cavity. I was reminded of the fact that my pelvis had never felt good throughout my entire life. My workout routine at this point was weight lifting. I was easily bench-pressing 135 lbs. and my upper body was defined as well as big. But my legs, even though I was squatting 115 lbs., wouldn't bulk up with strength or definition even over the three years that I lifted. My abdomen, no matter what exercises I did, would never get tight only bigger. I finally came to the realization that the sheath of abdominal muscle that separates during pregnancy never went back together after my daughter's birth 14 years before. There were two reasons for this muscle division: (1) my thyroid gland was running slow from birth and the thyroid gland dictates the muscles and tissues. (after the pregnancy during which I goitered, my thyroid didn't contain the energy to perform the task of bringing the sheath of abdominal muscle back together); and (2) the trauma of abandonment weakened this area emotionally which is probably why the hypothyroidism manifested its physical degeneration here. So now I had an abdomen, which was missing its natural corset. With only a few sessions of neurological emotional technique the charkas were healed, but my muscle would have to be mended back together.

Since 1987 I had experienced tremendous pain in my lower back and neck. Actually, within five years of the birth of my daughter my body was displaying symptoms of a skeletal breakdown. And by 1995 it was obvious that structural healing was the next step in my health quest knowing that the ground work had been laid by the healing of those charkas and my thyroid gland, although that work would not be done until 1996 before the reattachment of the muscle which is called a tummy tuck.

CHAPTER 16

Truth from Scriptures

My search took me to the book of I Corinthians: 12. I was familiar with these passages of Scripture because during the years spent in the ministry, we studied repeatedly the gift of the Holy Spirit and the gift ministries. God tells us once we have received the Holy Spirit that we can utilize the diversities of operations of the gift. And as verse 7 states, *"But the manifestation of the Spirit it is given to every man to profit withal."* The creator for our utilization has provided the proper tools so that we can come to enjoy abundant life, which would be the ultimate profit to us.

The operations of the gifts are listed in verses 8, 9, 10, and 11. Although all operations are equally important and available, I will focus on two, gifts of healings and working of miracles. As we follow chapter 12 verses 27 through 31, God has set some in the church to be workers of miracles and gifts of healing. So why not take advantage of this reality and truth and become empowered as God intended for us? By taking control of our own healthcare, we secure the responsibility and accountability of it and are responsible for the outcome of our health, good or bad. We make ultimate decisions for ourselves.

God has provided specific information for the carrying out of this responsibility.

In my search for truth, I found this information:

Another witness of early recommendations of colon hydrotherapy is the so-called Essene gospel of peace whose text dates from the 3rd century after Christ. The complete Aramatic manuscript exists in the secret archives of the Vatican, and a translation into old Slavonic is kept in the royal archives of the Hapsburgs, now the property of the republic of Austria.

We owe the existence of these two versions to the historian priests of the Essenes brotherhood who, under pressure of the advancing hoards of Genghis Khan, were forced to flee to the west, bearing all their ancient scriptures and icons.

It is to the merit of the International Biogenic Society of Matskee British Columbia, Canada, founded in 1928 by the philosopher Roman Rolan, Nobel Laureate of 1915, and Edmund Waldo Schecklee, a Hungarian bishop of the Unitarian church. Theologists have compared, edited and translated into English the old manuscripts.

During the more than 70 years since the publication of the translation of the ancient manuscripts, also known as the dead sea scrolls, more than 10 million readers have absorbed the message. Following is a condensed citation of the Essene gospel of peace:

Renew yourselves and fast for I tell you ⟨ uty that Satan and his plagues may only be cast out by fasting and by prayer. Go by yourself and fast alone and show your fasting to no man. The living God shall see it and great shall be your reward. And fast till Beelzebub and all these evils depart from you and all the angels of our earthly mother come and serve you. For I tell you truly unless you fast you shall never be free from the power of Satan and from all diseases that come from Satan. Fast and pray fervently seeking the power of the living God for your healing. While you fast, eschew the sins of man and seek our earthly mothers angels for he that seek shall find.

Seek the fresh air of the forest and of the fields and there in the midst of them shall you find the angel of air. Pull off your shoes and your clothing and suffer the angel of air to embrace all your body. Then breathe long and deeply that the angel of air may be brought within you. I tell you truly the angel of air shall cast out of your body all uncleanness, which defiled it without and within. And thus shall all evil smelling and unclean things rise out of you as the smoke of fire curls upwards and is lost in the sea of the air. For I tell you truly holy is the angel of air who cleanses all that is unclean and makes all evil smelling things of a sweet, sweet odor. No man may come before the face of God who the angel of air lets not pass. Truly, truly all must be born again by air and by truth for your body breathes the air of the earthly mother and your spirit breathes the truth of the heavenly father.

After the angel of air, seek the angel of water. Put off your shoes and your clothing and suffer the angel of water to embrace all your body. Cast yourself wholly into his enfolding arms and as often as you move the air with your breath, move with your body the water also. I tell you truly the angel of water shall cast out of your body all uncleanness, which defiled you without and within. And all unclean and evil smelling things shall flow out of you as the uncleanness of garments washed in water flow away and are lost in the stream of the river. I tell you truly holy is the angel of water who cleanses all that is unclean and makes all evil smelling things of a sweet odor. No man may come before the face of God whom the angel of water lets not pass. In your truth all must be born again of water and of truth. Your body bathes in the river of earthly life and your spirit bathes in the river of earthly life and your spirit bathes in the river of life everlasting. For you receive your blood from our earthly mother and the truth from our heavenly father think not that it is sufficient that the angel of water embrace you outwards only. I tell you truly the uncleanness within is greater by much than the uncleanness without. And he who cleanses himself without but within remains unclean is like two tones that outward are painted fair but are within full of all of *uncleanness and abominations so I tell you truly suffer the angel of water to baptize you also within that you may become free from all your past sins and that within likewise you may become as pure as the rivers foam scorching in the sunlight.*

Seek therefore a large trailing gourd having a stalk the length of a man. Take out its inwards and fill it with water from the river, which the sun has warmed. Hang it upon the branch of a tree and kneel upon the ground before the angel of water and suffer the end of the stalk of the trailing gourd to enter your hinder parts that the water may flow through all your bowels. Afterwards, rest kneeling on the ground before the angel of water and pray to the living God that he will forgive you all your past sins and pray the angel of water that he will free your body from every uncleanness and disease. Then let the water run out from your body that it may carry away from within it all the unclean and evil smelling things of Satan, and you shall see with your eyes and smell with your nose all the abominations and uncleanness which defiled the temple of your body. Even all the sins, which abide in your body tormenting you with all manner of pains. I tell you truly baptism with water frees you from all of these. Renew your baptizing with water on every day of your fast until the day when you see that the water, which flows out of you, is as pure as the river's foam. Then take your body to the coursing river and there in the arms of the angel of water render thanks

53

to the living God that he has freed you from your sins. And this holy baptizing by the angel of water is rebirth unto the new life. For your eyes shall henceforth see and your ears shall hear. Sin no more therefore after your baptism that the angels of air and of water may eternally abide in you and serve you evermore.

CHAPTER 17

1994 Environmental Clean-up

As the documentation of colonics show (see Chapter 19), I didn't stop after my bowel was clean in October 1993. My logic was to see what my body would do as I continued. Also I realized that if my body had been so full of old feces that it took 7 years to clean it up, and even though I'd come close to death's door, I still had been functioning with all that mess. Then even if I pushed the limits in the opposite direction, my body would let me know, and that's precisely what happened. My body totally rejected the water of the colonic during the beginning of the procedure where the water is introduced through the rectum. It took 7 years to get to the mucous lining of my colon and then my body protected itself. It was so obvious and I respected that, just as I respected the fact that it had been so dirty and wanted my logical self to clean it up. Now don't make the mistake of thinking that I'm the only person with this unique problem. All of our bodies are made of the same organic materials and all of us are eating the same inorganic processed foods. And we were not designed by God to eat processed food ever! That's why the body can't get rid of all of it. It's not real food! Think about this, if people were cleaning their bowels thousands of years ago when there was nothing but organic live food, then it's no wonder why it would take the average American many years of aggressive bowel management to get to a clean slate. I'm Proof! And I am not the only one!

Now I do need to address another subject. During the time between October of 1993 and January of 1995 at which time my body finally rejected the water. I cleansed my gallbladder, liver and pancreas. I obtained this information from various sources. The doctors doing the neurological Emotional Technique that Dr. Nicol studied with have a very good recipe for this and also Dr. Hulda Clark's books contain this vital information. They are very simple recipes that contain various combinations of foods and herbs that will gently but successfully flush the collected debris from your organs. Hundreds of bright green stones released from my body cavity! Also I did 3 or 4 consecutive flushes with a week in between each. This was aggressive but the proof was in the toilet each time hundreds of stones released. And remember I was having a colonic everyday at this point and my bowel was clean, so it was very obvious what everything was that came through the tube. It was very interesting that as I was cleansing my gallbladder and liver that my knees ballooned up for approximately 1 month! As those organs were busy cleaning up and detoxifying it affected my knees because it's these two organs that in fact do generate e knees also the shoulders, elbows, and ankles.

This information can be found in various Chinese medicine texts. I've grown intensely respectful toward the human body as I watched it work so perfectly during these years. And now that the bowel was clean these organs could with ease dump their waste where it was intended to go but really could not because my bowel had been so full previously. All the organs dump into the bowel but there has to be room otherwise the organ gets stuck holding onto the waste and you start having illness and disease, while the bowel also starts to respond in various ill ways.

CHAPTER 18

Last Environmental Parasite Clean-up

As I was finishing up with my environmental cleanup in 1995, I also had to face the fact that I probably had parasites! Interesting enough, because my bowel wasn't full of wonderful leftovers anymore, the smarter parasites (that hide out in the organs) that travel to the bowel to eat, attached themselves to the food, for fear of starvation! And they got swished out during the colonic. Threadworms!

The next parasite situation was the subject of nematodes. And this particular nematode was living in my pancreas with his family! It likely was there for many years, perhaps when I was a child. Keep in mind that my bowel is clean by this point, and many small symptoms have already disappeared by now, but these symptoms remained: My belly would swell when I walked near the energy of food or if I ate food. It would balloon up across the transverse colon where the liver, gallbladder, and pancreas set above. It affected my clothing and my husband said the never saw such a thing! Now I will say that every time I've needed health information for a particular situation, it's been provided. The diagnostic tool I chose to utilize again was contact reflex analysis, which determined that parasites were present in the pancreas. Also with the help of Dr. Nicol, we found a doctor who was teaching seminars on nematodes, and this information coincided with my symptoms. And also we learned the recipe for cleaning them out of the organ. We made a tincture with whiskey and marigold roots.

Now remember, while we're figuring this situation out I'm also doing liver and gallbladder flushes periodically along with a colonic each day. So as I'm doing a gallbladder and liver flush, Mr. Nematode must have been lunching in the wrong place and at the wrong time for him. Because of the gentle but forceful nature of the flushing process now transpiring within these organs, the nematode got flushed into the bowel and during the daily colonic a 7" flesh colored, plump nematode came through the tube. Myself and another individual saw it. She said, "Ooh, what was that? And I said, "What did it look like"? She replied, "an eel". Well interestingly enough the nickname of "eel." has been given to the nematode family by the health community. So now we have the tincture ready and for 1 week and a half I muscle-test for 6 shots each morning. Of course, the body's innate ability knew to use the tincture medicinally.

During this time period, my stomach ballooned up, like I was seven months pregnant. My pancreas was on fire; I could feel the heat with my hand. I also felt compelled to scratch, just like a scab that was healing. And then on August 26th, which just happened to be my birthday, the swelling subsided across my abdomen. The tension was gone and I felt very peaceful, very calm and almost blissful! AND VERY INTERESTINGLY "HOLY CRAP AGAIN!" The laboratory was fired up once again, as all the information and events proved their truths. Through these years I'm very certain that my liver, gallbladder, pancreas, and colon had been cleaned up very well and would work optimally. My internal hygiene was improving noticeably, as I never before in my life remembered feeling such a peaceful resource of energy. It was the ultimate high, non-toxic existence that I believe human beings are constantly searching for. NATURE'S FOUNTAIN OF YOUTH!

The ecological system exists. Parasites are part of it. They are real! Why not utilize your brain and the information readily available to educate yourselves as to how to live victoriously within the physical plane? People have for thousands of years dealt victoriously with these critters. If we're so smart, then why are they winning and so many of us dying from simple parasitical infections? This is the absolutely ridiculous price we pay for man's foolishness, denial and ignorance. We can go to the moon, but God forbid we're afraid to cleanse our wonderfully made bodies with a little water and remove some little creatures out of our precious bodies so that we can feel so good. Call me eccentric, but I'm in!

CHAPTER 19

Tummy Tuck, CST, Thyroid, Mouth

It is 1996, and by this time my colon is cleaned, my organs are clean and working quite well and the parasite activity is history. Many of my birth issues are settled also. I'm cruising!

I've decided to learn how to do the structural and emotional therapies now. I decided to study with Dr. John Upledger, my motive being this: He requires that you must actively participate in learning any procedures to achieve certification. So you are actively gaining your own health in order to practice as a healthcare professional. The healthcare professionals that are actively pursuing their own health are in my opinion much better qualified healthcare practitioners. They know what it takes to get healed, so they're much more sensitive and compassionate to others. But they also know when people are not serious about getting well, and wasting valuable time. So in July of 1996, I became certified as a Cranial Sacral Therapist, Level I. And in March 1997, I became certified in Cranial Sacral Therapy, Level II, and also received more personal healing during this time.

By this time, my thyroid gland was goitering. Do not think that because of extensive bowel management that this is why my thyroid goitered. I had classic hypothyroid symptoms all my life, as I listed earlier in my book. By now it was quite obvious and I felt like my gland was strangling me.

My neck was quite swollen. Also, my legs were edematous. At the suggestion of another healthcare practitioner, I used Atomidine, an organic iodine, from Edgar Casey's book. Within 2 weeks the edema was gone and my legs looked shapelier. Within 3 months my thyroid gland was healed. My heart, which had experienced stress (ANGINA PECTORIS) due to the weak thyroid gland, was quite peaceful now. My choice of diagnostic tool was the bio-energy machine, which revealed very low energy running in the thyroid gland and the heart. Also it was compromising the functioning of my other organs because the thyroid gland is a master gland and dictates your basal metabolic rate for your entire body. Within 3 months a second check on the bio-energy machine revealed increased energy in my thyroid gland and my heart totally balanced as it benefited from the thyroid gland's healing. This is a very important organ and I believe many Americans don't have healthy function of the thyroid gland. There are very few foods that feed the thyroid. These foods feed the thyroid gland; kelp, Irish moss, bladder wrack and dolce. Fish does contain iodine but only in salmon is the iodine already chelated to be received directly by the thyroid gland. Our foods in America don't contain these ingredients. And few people eat fish often enough in order to gain much benefit for the thyroid gland. That's why people that live near the sea and eat lots of fish are really healthy people, because they have healthy thyroid glands. And that gland is powerful in its role within the body. I believe because the diagnostic tools for thyroid testing have been proven to be very inadequate, that a very large portion of the population is experiencing many symptoms of hypothyroidism, and are not aware of it. And if the test doesn't show this information adequately, then people aren't getting what they need. Then healthcare can become very confusing. Remember this, the thyroid dictates the pituitary gland, adrenal glands and the hormonal glands directly, and controls the basal metabolic rate of your body.

Once my thyroid gland was healed, these very noticeable changes occurred within my body: I was no longer physically or mentally fatigued. It was like someone took the blinders off my eyes! Suddenly I could handle a lot more mentally with ease. My parotid glands weren't constantly swollen. My neck was no longer swollen. The edema was gone. The muscle controlling my bladder was much stronger. I was no longer constantly freezing, my body temperature adjusted accordingly. My cholesterol, which had been sky-high for many years, was normal now. I had a medical lab test showing my cholesterol to be very high previous to healing this gland and within six months a test showing my cholesterol to be normal. I've found information connecting hypothyroidism to high cholesterol. When the arteries become dehydrated from hypothyroidism, the liver will produce cholesterol and send it to the arteries to lubricate them. It is a protective mechanism. But because the predominant cause is never addressed (feeding the thyroid), the liver keeps producing more and more cholesterol and keeps sending it up to the arteries until the arteries get so clogged that the heart is compromised and stops. So the protective mechanism becomes the killer only because the bottom lying cause or source of the problem has been neglected. This information confirmed my healing process for my thyroid gland. The process of healing proved what information was true. Simple math! Also my blood pressure ran very low all my life, and I was always very thin. When the hypothyroidism progressed into advanced stages, I became overweight and my blood pressure was high. Now my blood pressure is normal. I'm in agreement with the healthcare community that believes any tissue and organ of the body can be regenerated with the proper procedures and organic substances. I am proof! And I'm not the only one. God created our bodies to live at least 1000 years since the garden and 250 years from Noah's day. There are cultures in the world today where people are very healthy well into their 100 years. But you'll only see that kind of health where physical plane principles have not been violated over and over again.

Documentation of Bowel Management:1987-1992

1987 – 1988 – 1989 – 1990 – 1991 – 1992
7 Day Colon Cleanse

Psyllium Seed	Bentonnite	Distilled Water	No Food	Green Magma	1 Coffee Enema
4x per day	4x per day	All Day	--	6 tablets, 4x per day	Per day

Followed this procedure every six months
from **1987** to July of **1992**.
1992 – July, August, September, October,
November, and December
1993 – January, February, March thru October

Apr. 1993	May 1993	June 1993	July 1993	Aug. 1993	Sept 1993	Oct. 1993	Nov. 1993	Dec. 1993
4/21	5/1	6/3	7/4	8/6	9/1	10/5	11/3	12/1
4/23	5/4	6/15	7/15	8/11	9/3	10/24	11/10	12/11
	5/7		7/16	8/15	9/8	*Colon Clean	11/15	12/12
	5/10		7/25	8/16	9/10		11/19	12/17
	5/14		7/27	8/17	9/23		11/29	12/22
	5/17			8/18	9/27			12/23
	5/20			8/20	9/28			12/24
	5/22							12/25
	5/24							
	5/27							

Approximately 100 colonics with the documentation of each colonic from this point on.

January 1994	February 1994	March 1994	April 1994	May 1994	June 1994
1/6	2/1	3/1	4/1	5/4	6/5
1/7	2/3	3/3	4/5	5/5	6/7
1/8	2/9	3/4	4/11	5/11	6/8
1/10	2/14	3/10	4/19	5/12	6/9
1/12	2/19	3/11	4/21	5/14	6/10
1/13	2/25	3/18	4/22	5/20	6/17
1/15		3/23	4/23	5/25	6/21
1/17		3/27	4/24	5/31	6/25
1/20			4/25		6/27
1/27			4/26		
1/29			4/28		

July 1994	Aug. 1994	Sept. 1994	Oct. 1994	Nov. 1994	Dec. 1994
7/3	8/1	9/2	10/2	11/1	12/4
7/7	8/2	9/3	10/3	11/2	12/6
7/11	8/3	9/4	10/4	11/3	12/8
7/12	8/4	9/5	10/5	11/4	12/10
7/13	8/5	9/6	10/6	11/5	12/12
7/14	8/6	9/7	10/7	11/6	12/14
7/15	8/7	9/8	10/8	11/7	12/15
7/17	8/8	9/11	10/9	11/8	12/16
7/20	8/9	9/12	10/10	11/9	12/18
7/21	8/10	9/13	10/11	11/10	12/19
7/23	8/11	9/14	10/12	11/12	12/22
7/24	8/12	9/21	10/13	11/13	12/23
7/25	8/13	9/23	10/14	11/17	12/25
7/26	8/14	9/24	10/15	11/18	12/28
7/27	8/15	9/26	10/16	11/21	12/30
7/28	8/16	9/27	10/18	11/22	12/31
7/29	8/17	9/28	10/19	11/24	
7/30	8/1	9/29	10/20	11/27	
7/31	8/21	9/30	10/23	11/29	
	8/22		10/24		
	8/23		10/25		
	8/25		10/26		
	8/26		10/27		
	8/27		10/28		
	8/28		10/29		
	8/29		10/30		
	8/31		10/31		

January 1995	February 1995	March 1995	April 1995	May 1995	June 1995
1/2	2/2	3/10	4/1	5/20	6/4
1/6	2/4	3/16	4/7	5/24	6/6
1/7	2/5	3/20	4/9	5/28	6/12
1/9	2/6	3/21	4/17		6/24
1/10	2/6	3/25	4/21		
1/11	2/8		4/22		
1/12	2/12		4/23		
1/13	2/13		4/26		
1/14			4/29		
1/15					
1/16					
1/18					
1/19					
1/23					
1/24					
1/25					
1/26					
1/27					

July 1995	Aug. 1995	Sept. 1995	Oct. 1995	Nov. 1995	Dec. 1995
7/9	8/7	9/6	10/3	11/2	12/11
7/16	8/16	9/15	10/6	11/10	12/19
7/25	8/22	9/20	10/11	11/17	12/27
7/29	8/28	9/22	10/17	11/23	
		9/23	10/26		

71

January 1996	February 1996	March 1996	April 1996	May 1996	June 1996
1/6	2/2	3/7		5/16	6/10
1/11	2/10	3/16		5/25	6/21
1/21	2/16	3/27			
1/26	2/23				

July 1996	August 1996	September 1996	October 1996	November 1996	December 1996
7/22	8/29	9/4	10/4	11/4	12/26
			10/28	11/30	

January 1997	February 1997	March 1997	April 1997	May 1997	June 1997
1/19	2/9	3/3	4/3	5/2	6/4
		3/15	4/5	5/5	6/8
		3/21	4/8	5/8	6/11
		3/25	4/12	5/11	6/15
		3/28	4/16	5/14	6/19
		3/31	4/19	5/17	6/22
			4/23	5/18	6/25
			4/25	5/25	6/29
			4/28	5/28	
				5/31	

July 1997	August 1997	September 1997	October 1997	November 1997	December 1997
7/4	8/1	9/1	10/1	11/1	12/8
7/7	8/5	9/4	10/3	11/8	12/14
7/10	8/8	9/7	10/6	11/17	12/22
7/15	8/11	9/14	10/10	11/28	12/30
7/18	8/15	9/16	10/17		
7/21	8/18	9/21	10/26		
7/23	8/21	9/25			
	8/24	9/28			
	8/28				

January 1998	February 1998	March 1998	April 1998	May 1998	June 1998
1/8	2/1	3/4	4/16	5/1	6/1
1/26	2/7	3/10	4/23	5/8	6/7
	2/16	3/19		5/14	6/14
	2/25	3/29		5/22	6/21
					6/28

July 1998	August 1998	Sept. 1998	Oct. 1998	Nov. 1998	Dec. 1998
7/4	8/2	9/5	10/4	11/10	12/7
7/12	8/9	9/13	10/13	11/16	12/14
7/22	8/16	9/20	10/19	11/24	12/21
7/28	8/24	9/27	10/26	11/30	12/27
	8/31		10/31		

January 1999	February 1999	March 1999	April 1999	May 1999	June 1999
1/6	2/9	3/1	4/5	5/3	6/8
1/11	2/12	3/7	4/11	5/16	
1/18	2/22	3/21	4/20	5/23	
1/20		3/29	4/26	5/31	
1/31					

July 1999	Aug. 1999	Sept. 1999	Oct. 1999	Nov. 1999	Dec. 1999
7/3	8/8	9/2	10/11	11/3	12/1
7/30		9/22	10/28	11/19	12/15
				11/28	12/20

January 2000	February 2000	March 2000
1/1	2/8	3/8
1/3 *103° temperature		
1/4 Fever completely gone within 8 hrs.		
1/21		

CHAPTER 20

Tummy Tuck April Fools' Day 1996

It was time to address the abdominal muscle, an obvious distended lower abdominal problem. No matter how much I worked those muscles, my abdomen got bigger. I felt like I looked like a much older woman and my posture was very poor. My torso was collapsed. I had no balance. I still had lower back pain caused by a weak abdominal cavity. My thyroid was healed, so I knew my body would be capable of maintaining the corrected muscle activity in that area. Also those 2nd and 3rd charkas issues had healed, so now I felt it was time to surgically have my sheath of muscle restored to normalcy, to complete the total recovery process in that area of my body. I interviewed several doctors in the Nashville area. I had four consultations with Dr. Blalock over a period of 8 months. I observed that he displayed great integrity, sensitivity and respect for the human body. I hired him for this job. So on April Fools' Day, which happened to be a Monday, I was his first client of the day. Upon awakening, I could feel a sense of strength in my abdominal area, almost like a sense of being complete. My recovery from the surgery was swift. I took large quantities of organic complexes consisting of amino acids, thyroid foods, raw bananas and oranges to stimulate my immune system, and good organic power drinks. My body was healing so fast that I could literally feel the heat from the healing process. I also made sure that I was eliminating the narcotics from my liver and kidneys by doing several colonics within the two weeks of surgery. Literally, fluorescent green narcotics that smelled like narcotics left my body cavity. Colonics proved to be a beneficial tool used as a post surgery modality.

Although that part of the surgery healed quickly, I noticed within 2 years that my abdomen was numb. Of course that's one of the consequences on the list of side affects of this surgery. As I'd been quite confident that I received permission from my higher power to do this surgery, I was also confident that further information would lead me to further healing in this situation. In 1998 a neuromuscular therapist came into my office for colonics. After talking with her about my abdomen, I decided that she was the therapist for me. I had a 11/2-hour session with her every week for one year straight. Here again I utilized the truths I'd learned throughout the last decade: To do what it takes to secure results, not what you may think it will take. Let the truth unfold and dictate the pace. Once I obtained magnificent results, I cut back to 11/2-hours, 2x a month.

Remember, when traumas change the function of the body cavity for many years, once something is fixed, there are other things that must be reworked back to normalcy, because the body is compensating. So with that truth in mind we continued to work the muscles and tissues back to the correction. My hips had been locked up for over six months; I couldn't lie on my back. In one visit she corrected that problem. I couldn't feel my fingers on my abdomen. She released the tissue and reconnected the flow of energy to the nerve endings, I could feel the lightest touch on my abdomen once again. My bladder muscle within those two years had become weak, and I was starting to leak with a sneeze. But slowly I saw a change in my deep tissue circulation, which resulted with change in that area. She also released the scar tissue right in the scar, so that the scar itself doesn't cause unevenness in that area. And these therapies are available to anyone that would like to utilize them. They're excellent for post-surgery situations. It's very important to thoroughly explore all information in order to obtain the total benefit in any health situation. I'm eternally grateful to this therapist for the personal integrity she possesses in her life and work, and for the high standard of truth she maintains in her life. That's why I was blessed to have obtained the full reward of my labor so that all will be well with me and I may travel further into the more-than-abundant life.

CHAPTER 21

Mercury Poisoning

It is late 1996, and my bowel is clean, the parasites gone, the birth traumas healed, the tummy muscle restored and the thyroid healed. My biography has been changed and now my biology has been restored like new, not even like when I was a child. Better! Of course, my body basically resembles the body I've always had. My legs, which developed immaturely and would never develop muscle no matter what I did, now with the added help of practicing yoga, are developing muscles and strength that I've never experienced before. My pelvis is dynamically strong. I could never stand for any length of time, but now I can stand forever without becoming tired. My collapsed torso is regenerated and now my posture is strong and upright. My walk is tireless. I actually grew taller. My spinal column is perfectly restored and does not house toxins anymore, because my liver and colon are clean. We degenerate so rapidly that I have actually regenerated and regained my youth.

And now through a period of a year, during 1996 into 1997, I decided to bring my healing process to its final culmination. It was time to remove the 10 dental fillings. After doing much research throughout this decade, I understood the bottom-lying cause of disease in the physical plane is poison. I'd cleaned up my environment relating to food, skin lotions, hair products, laundry soaps, bath soaps, and toothpaste -- anything that would re-pollute my clean body. Now it was time to remove from my mouth the horrendous poison put there without my permission. My parents were ignorant and trusted in the laws they believed were made to protect them. Many Americans believed that it was safe to put mercury and many other various types of metals in your mouth as fillings. They were misled! Many books have been written with much evidence like my own story about the swift deterioration of health that proceedes this dental work.

In 1996 in Nashville, I knew of no one in the healthcare or dental fields that knew anything concerning this dilemma. So, I figured if I'd saved my life up to this point because I understood the systems and organs and how to keep my environment clean that I probably stood a good chance of figuring out how to chelate the mercury and other metals through my blood stream and out my rectum once and for all. And that's exactly what I did! Once the fillings were replaced, I noticed my gums and teeth were sore and sensitive to heat and cold. And it never got better! Now you may think if I had used the Huggins method, that that may not have occurred. But I've observed many people personally that have done the same dental procedures with the Huggins method and are experiencing the same problems. No tool or piece of equipment will ever be able to stop the mercury from releasing into the bloodstream at the base of the tooth where it meets the gum, although, I'm sure the Huggins method probably reduces the amount of mercury that may escape in other ways! Remember, small amounts of mercury are deadly, no matter what your dentist may tell you.

No other symptoms other than the sensitivity of my teeth and gums were occurring initially. But over the next 2 to 3 years I started to gain weight. Now remember, I was living a meticulous lifestyle! My skin tissue was turning from feeling like (clay) and easily being sculpted to feeling like rubber and not being able to be moved. My lymphatic system drained as a result of having bodywork, but within a day it would be full with liquid again. I actually felt like I was suffocating to death! As time progressed, my heart once again was becoming stressed, as I was starting to have panic attacks. And my weight gain was moving from 125 lbs. steadily up to 170 lbs. over the course of 3 years. I also continuously felt heat coming off my body, especially from my palms and the bottoms of my feet, not like a fever, but heat much like the heat felt when toxins are coming through the colonic tube. I was determined to receive the pertinent information. And I did! I just asked for wisdom and guidance and both were literally laid at my feet. As I made a mental evaluation of recent events that may have introduced pollutants into my body cavity, I remembered the removal of my mercury fillings. This information also warned of the devastating effects that may occur as a result of having them removed especially in relationship to pregnancy, which was something we'd been contemplating at this time. I decided to heed that warning. So by this time my head felt like it was going to blow off my shoulders! My choice of diagnostic tool was iridology. I needed help. The wonderful ancient diagnostic tool of iridology proved to be very helpful. My eyes showed that my bloodstream was full of mercury and that yeast was magnetized to it. The sodium I was receiving from a packaged organic vegetable protein drink wasn't being absorbed by my small intestine. The sodium was being thrown back into my blood stream and was multiplying to levels harmful to my heart The mercury was inhibiting the processing and the absorption of nutrients in the small intestine. These symptoms are related to Celiac's disease.

At this time, I've eliminated all gluten from my diet, only eating 2 eggs with salad for lunch and salmon and salad for dinner. Eating pineapple throughout the day, I was having absolutely no food cravings. The kidneys and liver were also being affected. Because I was doing 1 colonic per week at this time, the liver was holding up quite well, showing only signs of heat flashes. But the kidneys were stressed out between the mercury and the yeast. I was urinating every 5 minutes and could see the yeast in the urine. I really do believe colonics saved my life in this situation. My body would have given out without that release. But I was obviously running out of time. I read some information about natural vegetable glycerin and its unique properties. What grabbed my attention was that this product is the only substance known with the ability to dissolve the inorganic compounds that have accumulated in the tissue and carry this toxic residue away as waste. The glycerin is the only known substance that can achieve this process in areas that are so small that only one blood cell can pass through a blood vessel at a time. It sounded like what was happening to me. Glycerin is an important intermediate in the metabolism of carbohydrates and fats. Without the important process of metabolism, these carbohydrates and fats can coagulate and form a plaque of all sorts in various parts of the body, causing all manner of depository and circulatory problems. I just found the source that would chelate the mercury and yeast through my circulatory system into my lungs, liver, and kidneys. Followed with colonics that would then remove the waste out of the body cavity. And that's exactly what happened! I took 2 tablespoons per day of glycerin and 2 capsules with each meal of Kantitta, a product consisting of condurango bark, red clover and yellow dock. This product cleaned the yeast out of my bloodstream. I started doing this procedure eve day in June of 1999. The weight started to melt losing 2 lbs. per 15 days. I also took Co Q enzyme immediately to support my heart and within 24 hrs,. my heart was stabilizing. By Christmas of 1999, I was at 143 lbs. and starting to look and feel like me again! My skin was returning to normal and was no longer like rubber. My lymphatic system was staying drained and my neck was not holding fluid because my kidneys were less stressed. My body was displaying wonderful detox symptoms. I was eliminating through my nose and sinus cavity long green colored strings of thick yeasty mucous. For 1 month solid, this debris came from the deepest cavities in my body. And I continued to do 1 colonic per week until the small intestine was working better and little waste was eliminating through the colonic. Then I cut back to 2 colonics per month. Remember I am also having 2 to 3 bowel movements per day. So I'm releasing large amounts of debris from my body cavity continuously through these months.

In March 2000, my body wouldn't drop below 143 lbs. I decided that 1 day a week I'd eat only high enzymatic fruit, watermelon, papaya and pineapple, maintaining my usual diet on the other 6 days. After the second day on the second week of doing this, I dropped to 138 lbs. But my body had to fever for this to transpire. It seemed the enzymatic fruit caused the still-toxic fatty tissue to release more of the mercury and yeast. Again my sinus cavities were releasing more sludge from the depths of my body cavity, which caused my body to fever in order to burn the debris. I felt like my body was purging on a cellular basis. Our bodies are magnificent instruments when we help them honestly.

This narrative brings my healing process current. And "holy crap" is just that -- "holy". Don't ever underestimate the effect and the power that our elimination holds in your life! God is in the driver's seat and is the divine artist, not man.

CHAPTER 22

Vegetable Glycerin vs. Alcohol

The natural vegetable glycerin used as a base for the extraction process of an herb or plant is unsurpassed. The glycerin, being a hygroscopic liquid and a trihydric alcohol, gives this substance the ability to extract the water-soluble nutrients and the oils from the herbs, thus making a complete herbal extract with all the plant residue factors (prf's).

Natural vegetable glycerin is a trihydric alcohol (a type of alcohol that has none of the negative effects of regular alcohol), forming alcoholates, esters and numerous healthful derivatives. This substance has the ability to dissolve and put in solution not only organic minerals but also inorganic minerals. Making glycerin a most valuable substance for the extraction process. While being the carrier for the extraction of organic substances out of herbs to the cell level, the glycerin has the ability to dissolve the inorganic compounds that have accumulated in the tissue and carry this toxic residue away as waste. The glycerin is the only known substance that can achieve this process in areas that are so small that only one blood cell can pass through a blood vessel at a time.

Glycerin is an important intermediate in the metabolism of carbohydrates and fats. Without the important process of metabolism, these carbohydrates and fats can coagulate and form a plaque of sorts in various parts of the body, causing all manner of depository and circulatory problems.

ALCOHOL

Alcohol used as an extracting agent of herbs is most inferior. The alcohol will cause more harm than good, in that it takes away most every nutrient upon which the body is dependent. Alcohol usually runs between 20 and 70 percent in alcohol extracts. Alcohol also causes cancer, dyspepsia, epilepsy, gastritis, gout, hay fever, headaches, heart disease, hyperthyroidism, prostatitis, poor sexual desires, ulcers, and liver damage and B-Complex deficiency.

Alcohol causes the brain to become oxygen-starved, causing the entire body to become dehydrated. The Busy Bee Publication – March 1999, Issue 45, Honeycomb Industries

CHAPTER 22

Basic Facts: Colon Hygiene and the Body

I suppose some simple facts about the functioning of our bowel may help to establish the desire in individuals to do some bowel cleansing. First, the whole digestive tract is legally an external organ, which means it's necessary to clean it, it's just like your mouth, teeth, ears, and nose. And you know how you feel when you don't take the time to perform those simple tasks. It also means that you have the right to clean your bowel. This is not a medical procedure, but a hygiene procedure and it's your body, so it's your right religiously and constitutionally! Even though colon hygiene is in the hygiene category, I do believe it's the absence of performing these simple hygienic practices that has opened us up as a nation to the volatile state of disease that we're in fact witnessing.

The bowel was divinely designed to work based upon stimulation. When you're chewing food, if it's a live food, the digestion process that starts in the mouth will begin to stimulate your peristalsis, which is the motion of the bowel to defecate; this signals your feet to carry you to a toilet. It's important to remember that the food has to contain organic substances.

The bowel can't be stimulated by packaged dead food, and that's why people don't cramp in the abdominal area. Their peristaltic action becomes lazy and the proportion of food that goes in compared to what is released is way out of line. This is why herbal bowel cleansers are necessary. Many years ago, a person would eat throughout the day fennel, flaxseed, peppermint, sienna, cascara sagrada cactus, aloe, etc. as part of their normal diets. So they had no problem eliminating. Also, if you don't cramp, you'll not eliminate. The body was designed to cramp when the perasalsis is in motion. I don't understand the negative connotations associated with abdominal cramping occurring as warning labels on products. When I cramp I know I'll be feeling fabulous after the bowel movement! It does not scare me to cramp and then eliminate. I understand my bowel process. By the way, it's the live enzymes contained in live food that are needed for the elimination process.

During the processing of food the destruction of these enzymes does have a devastating effect on the elimination process. Because it is these enzymes, contained in the uncooked foods, that keep the balance of harmful bacteria and spores from all different types of parasites balanced and under control.

The enzymes are like Pac men; they eat up debris and garbage! So it may be necessary and beneficial for the average American to get a good dose of enzymes from an organic supplement these days.

CHAPTER 23

Various Cleansing Products

An important topic for discussion is the quality of various bowel cleansing products and the effects they each have on the bowel. Over the last 14 years I've used them all and through experimentation know what they'll do in the digestive tract. Psyllium is 100% indigestible and is a bulking agent, just as the label states. This product I used only when I fasted for 7 days. It was sweeping feces through but it was absolutely necessary to pull it all out through the rectum or the psyllium would re-harden inside the colon and cause more problems within the bowel. Psyllium will bulk up the already-bulked up processed feces and your bowel will be in worse condition than before. I've witnessed many people that have taken just plain psyllium, thinking it would be the fiber to help their bowel work better, but found that it totally stopped their bowel movements and made their bellies balloon. The only fiber that we absolutely need is fiber found in fruits and vegetables and herbal cleansers. Because this type of fiber has the ability to explode the already-bulked up, hardened feces and will prepare the old feces to be in a better form in order that the bowel can then expel them through the rectum. We don't have textbook bodies in this century. We've evolved into polluted cesspools, ded with everything that's in opposition to we need to be healthy. Just as John Robbins states in his book, *"Diet For A New America"*, each American is carrying around several pounds of pollutant from various sources. It's legal to buy poison in foods and drinks in any grocery store. Open your eyes and ears to the truth and the real reality that exists today in America. We must initiate aggressive removal of this junk in order to get back to the textbook bodies we think we have. We've come into a whole new set of health challenges now and that's environmental illness. That is why the methods that have been somewhat helpful in the past no longer work, but are contributing to the breakdown of the human body. The livers in America can't take one more dose of poison from anything, even legal drugs. People in this country are very ill, walking time bombs, because everybody's afraid to acknowledge that we've been stupid enough to allow ourselves to be poisoned and actually are willing to pay someone to do it to us!

Remember that the truth from the DIVINE is not synonymous with American culture. Man's wisdom is foolishness to God. That's why we're foolishly and needlessly dying.

Ephesians 4: 17, 18, 19 states: *This I say therefore, and testify in the Lord, that ye henceforth walk not as other Gentiles walk, in the vanity of their mind. Having the understanding darkened, being alienated from the life of God through the ignorance that is in them, because of the blindness of their heart; Who being past feeling have given themselves over unto lasciviousness, to work all uncleanness with greediness.*

You may want to claim your inheritance; it's yours for the asking and then the executing of the principles.

Remember also that we're body, soul and spirit! The real body and soul parts of our lives are undernourished. For some reason we think spirituality is proven by studying the word and reading it, praying and talking about it, or how often we show up at church. In the meantime, as we are so busy doing these things, we forget to take time to prepare our meals properly. We aren't able to find the time to selectively grocery shop or to be still long enough to listen to our bodies when they're longing for rest and relaxation or begging us to remove these poisons out of it and truly not nourishing or caring for our bodies in a divine fashion. But true spirituality lies in the nourishment of all three sides, learning to say "no" to man and "yes" to the divine plan, traveling out of the martyring love into the true love of self. Then you will truly understand what's involved in loving and actually helping other human beings to live and travel further into truth.

Dr. Wood designed the "gravity flow" method. The procedure is absolutely safe. I've never seen any negative results from this procedure.

Colonics will only reveal health crisis already presently occurring within the body. It's NEVER better for the body to hold waste than to discard it. If you stay within the guidelines of this procedure, you'll only travel into wellness. Remember, we travel away from wellness into disease. So if we begin to clean up our environment before we have a disease, we'll not get a disease. So why wait until you have a major illness to start cleaning your bowel? This is just pure and simple logic. Also it's important to understand that anyone who hasn't had a colonic or done at least 15 colonics within a 25-day period is not a valid source of information. It's a sad reality that healthcare practitioners can only take their clients as far as they've gone themselves. It's not good for a healthcare practitioner to limit another human being in their health quest, especially when you've committed your life to serving your fellow-human being in health. And your ignorance may not be a sufficient excuse especially when the information is certainly available and obtainable. As healthcare professionals we're accountable for those actions. If you've never had colonics, then you can only advise others to check it out for themselves and draw their own conclusions. You shouldn't draw any conclusions about something you've never done, regardless what information you've read or how much schooling you've had. The experts in colon hygiene are the people themselves that have put in the time and energy, and therefore have discovered the benefits and obtained the information from experiences.

The mathematical concept for health is simply subtraction!